Stop Losing Sleep

Establish Healthy Sleep Patterns to Improve your Health and Energy

By Kyle Richards

Table of Contents

Introduction

It is my hope that this will inspire you to learn more about the topic of sleep and find some real, practical solutions for the best quality of sleep you can get, for both yourself and your family.

It seems most of the population struggles, or will struggle with various sleep issues, at some point in their lives. The root problem can be different for each individual, so it's important to find what works for you.

As one who does have a sleep disorder, called sleep apnea, I know firsthand how sleep issues can greatly disrupt a person's life. Don't hesitate to seek medical help from a sleep clinic if you need it, it can be life changing!

Kyle Richards

In this book you'll find useful information on sleep in general, its importance, and many strategies to try at home to improve your sleep quality (many applicable to children & teens as well), thus improving your health overall and energy levels. Keep reading.

Why are we Having Trouble Sleeping?

"Death, so called, is a thing which makes men weep. And yet a third of life is passed in sleep." –George Gordon Byron.

This reference is a wake-up call to the people of this fast paced era, to take sleeping seriously as a vital component of our existence. It is sounding an alarm for everyone to stop their fast paced lifestyles, and rethink the importance of sleep in our lives.

Sleep, though seemingly passive, is a very vibrant activity (as proven by EEG readings that show brain waves during sleep are similar to the brain waves during wakefulness). It is as significant as daily activities of living, like self-care habits, work and play. But unlike hobbies, sleep can easily mean the difference between productivity and slacking off, a healthy body and a diseased one, and a ticket to longevity or a trip to the hospital. It directly affects every aspect of our lives like our moods, social engagements, behaviors, attitudes, and even our personal aspirations.

What is the problem?

Nowadays, a large portion of the population are actually sleep deprived. The problem of sleep deprivation, is defined as a person's lack of sleep, due to the lack of opportunity, or time to sleep because of intentional decisions and priorities. If you are not convinced, here is a quick check: Think about your sleep last night. How many hours did you sleep? According to the National Sleep Foundation and the National Institute of Health, an adult must spend an average of 7-8 hours on a good night's sleep. What's your number?

According to the 2014 National Health Interview Survey in the US, almost 30% of the adults reported an average of less than 6 hours of sleep a day in 2005-2007. About 38% of the adults in the study, reported unintentionally falling asleep during the day for at least one day in a 30 day period.

Why is it a serious problem?

Sleep promotes productivity and enables the renewal of the mind and body. Simply stated, we are refreshed by sleeping. With less sleep, people are more prone to sickness and accidents, both in the workplace and on the road. Sleep deprivation is a public safety and health concern. People who have insufficient sleep are more likely to suffer from chronic diseases. Significantly, about 50-70 million adults in the US are experiencing sleep or wakefulness disorders. This is according to the study made by the Institute of Medicine in Washington, DC.

What is the cause of the problem?

The pressing problem of sleep deprivation and its consequences, grows out of shifting interests or other factors. As our era is progressing with technological breakthroughs in the form of industrial machinery, gadgets, and up-to-date computer programs that make life more convenient and interesting for today's generation, we now have very different priorities compared to that of previous eras.   After all, new technology means new career opportunities. More people are making careers out of these newly available options. For example, with the growing popularity of outsourcing as a means of availing of services while cutting costs, and more corporations become global, employees in different time zones adapt to the work shift of other time zones as necessary.

Also, new technology means new ways for entertainment. The 'selfie' generation which has sprouted out of the ideals of self promotion, motivates individuals from all walks of life to take more taxing career choices in order to afford new comforts that are new and personally fulfilling. Sometimes with the increases in living costs, extra part time work or overtime is necessary just to make ends meet. Losing a few hours of sleep for a few steps up the career ladder? This is nothing new; it has become commonplace in this era.

And so we reap the consequences. Ironically, the very gadgets we so enjoy, have been shown to distract our brains from sleeping. This is according to the study released by the National Sleep Foundation in 2011. According to the statistics, 95% of Americans use electronics an hour before bedtime. Researchers hypothesize that the use of electronics exposes them to light and distractive activity, which delays the onset of sleep that results in sleep deprivation. Interestingly, 60% of the people in the same study claim that they are experiencing sleep problems, and have not had enough sleep during the week. 85% say that it affects their mood, 72% say it affects their family life and responsibilities in the home, and 68% say it affects their social lives.

The damaging habit of not sleeping well (and not minding it) is also setting up a wrong example for the younger generation, who are also beginning to reap the consequences. Here is an example: In a household, if the father or the mother habitually sleeps after midnight because of work or television, the other members of the family see these actions as the norm, and tend to follow them. Even if parents do enforce reasonable bedtimes for children, the kids see something else modeled.

What can we do about it?

We must realize now that sleep deprivation is a serious problem. By knowledge, we change our actions, and by modifying our actions, we can develop new habits, and in time, we develop healthier behaviors.

Perhaps we feel that we are doing right for ourselves by prioritizing career advancements and night pleasures like clubbing and nightcaps, which are also products of our changing culture. But truthfully, it is costing us more than what we perceive. By putting sleep in the backseat of our priorities, we are setting ourselves up for long term health risks and sudden accidents.

History About Sleep

"Even a soul submerged in sleep is hard at work and helps make something of the world." -Heraclitus, *Fragments*

Definition of Sleep

Sleep is a complex and active process of physiological restoration. It is the condition of the body and mind in which the nervous system is in a restorative mode; the eyes are closed, and consciousness is temporarily suspended. It naturally occurs as a state of altered consciousness, in which there is a decreased ability to react to external stimuli. In this condition, activities of the senses are inhibited, and almost all of the voluntary muscles are inactive.

Sleep is a biological state of rest. During sleep, the brain stays active while most of the body's organ systems are in a state of increased repair and maintenance at the cellular level. It is an established biological need. About one-third of our existence consists of sleep. It is essential for maintaining productivity throughout the day. Without restorative sleep, a person cannot learn, create, and communicate at the optimal level. A few skips of a good night's rest can cause substantial stress for the body, which can potentially lead to a major mental and physical breakdown.

History and Background of Sleep

Long before research established scientific facts about it, sleep was considered to be a passive state in which the brain becomes "inactive" or "switched off". Throughout history, sleep patterns and ideas pertaining to it have evolved, but the need for this "sweet balm" that soothes and restores our body after a long day of work and play has not changed. To this day, many sleep scientists are still studying and making sense of the mystery of this process. There are still a lot of gray areas in the field of sleep, but observations and studies made throughout history have nevertheless contributed to further understanding the inner workings of the body during this significant biological process.

In 600-800 B.C., segmented sleep was largely the norm for centuries. This means that two sleep periods in a day was common, and it was a period of prayer, thinking, reflecting on dreams, drinking ale, and visiting neighbors at night. Of the first sleeping period Homer wrote, "In his first sleep, call up your hardiest cheer."

In 450-500 B.C., the earliest documented sleep theory was written by Alcmaeon. He stated that sleep was a loss of consciousness which occurred when blood drained from the vessels on the body surface. His study resulted in further observation and experimentation about sleep.

Around 400 B.C., a new theory was suggested that bodies tend to feel cool to the touch when people sleep as blood goes to the inner regions of the body. This was recorded in Corpus Hippocraticum, a collection of medical writings largely attributed to Hippocrates. Also, the concept of circadian rhythm, an internally controlled body process that repeats itself every 24 hours, was first recorded by Androsthenes, the scribe of Alexander the Great.

In 350 B.C., sleep was viewed as a necessary time of physical recovery. Aristotle theorized that sleep was caused directly by warm vapors rising from the stomach to the heart, which was believed at that time to be the organ that controls consciousness. This was also the reason used to explain why people feel sleepy after having a meal.

Around 162 A.D., it was discovered that consciousness was controlled by the brain. Galen experimented on the brain and refuted Aristotle's claim.

In 1584, Aristotle's theory that warm vapors from the stomach rising to the heart during digestion that caused sleep, was promoted by Thomas Cogan in his book, 'The Haven of Health'. He suggested that meat, milk, and wine produced a lot of these "warm vapors" more readily than any other food items.

In the Renaissance era, theories related to sleep and wakefulness began to emerge. Some scientists and philosophers believed that sleep was caused by oxygen or blood deprivation in the brain. Others believed that toxins build up in the body during the state of wakefulness, and then get flushed out during sleep. Still others thought it was an inhibitory reflex that shut off the body and caused sleep.

During the Age of Enlightenment, dreams were viewed as significant and sacred. Interpretation and recording of dreams became a trend especially among the intellectual class. Alfred Maury and Marquis d'Hervey de Saint-Denis were prominent among those who recorded their dreams daily, studied them and interpreted them.

In the Industrial Age, the bedroom was regarded as a strictly personal area. Also, sleeping beyond seven to eight hours a day was viewed negatively as lazy.

In the 1900s, scientists began to discover that the brain; not the sun or stomach gases, controlled sleep and wakefulness. The science of sleep medicine was also born. In 1939, Nathaniel Kleitman published recordings of his years of investigative and experimental research in

Sleep and Wakefulness, which is regarded as a milestone in the study of sleep.

In 1970, the first sleep center (the laboratory where studies of sleep and diagnoses of sleep disorders can be properly conducted) was established at Stanford University. The Association of Sleep Disorders was also founded. In 1983, studies made by Allan Rechtschaffen and his colleagues revealed that sleep deprivation results in serious health problems and even death. The importance of sleep is being highlighted by many studies. Even so, many people in this decade find it difficult to manage their hectic schedules to accommodate enough sleep time to recover properly from their daily lives.

Kyle Richards

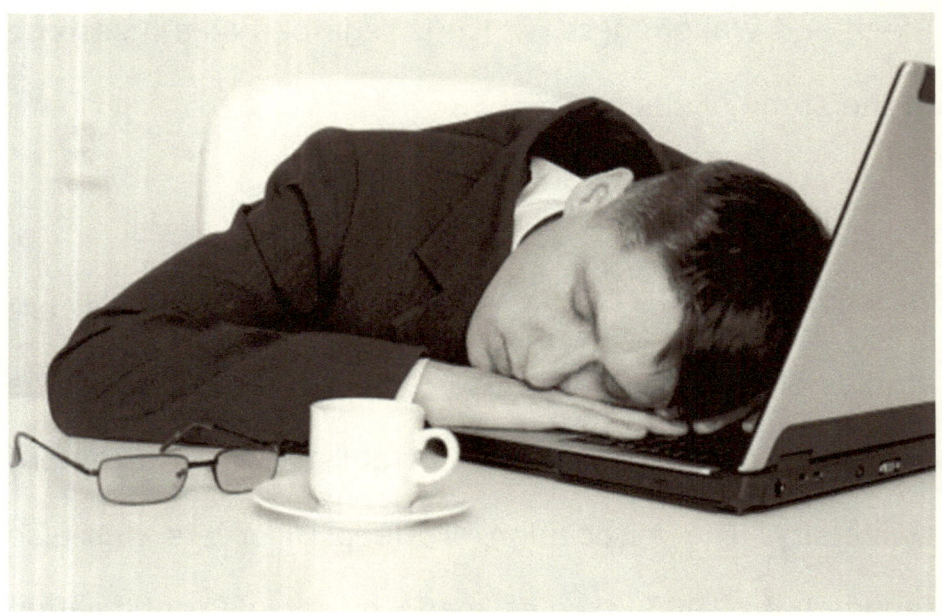

Importance of Sleep

Why is sleep so important to us? Sleep is needed to achieve and maintain overall productivity and holistic health. It rejuvenates the immune, nervous, skeletal, and muscular systems. Losing a few good hours of it, can cause unnecessary stress to the body.

Sleep deprivation is a serious concern for public safety every day, at work and on the road. With inhibited sensitivity to external stimuli, a person can sustain unnecessary accidents both on the job, and while driving.

Generally, when people sleep less than they should, they have mental blanks more often and are more forgetful, get sick more often due to decreased immune response (thus making them more vulnerable to certain diseases), more at risk of depression and diabetes, more prone to obesity, have difficulty focusing on regular tasks, easily fatigued, experience increased sensitivity to pain and various environmental stressors, such as noise or work overload. Even mundane tasks of daily living and decision making becomes challenging for them, requiring much more effort to accomplish. They also may have impaired moral judgment and in severe cases, might experience hallucinations.

A person who lacks sleep and drinks alcohol, will noticeably have a lower tolerance to it, because the body tends to metabolize alcohol less effectively when it is not well rested.

Physiologically, the normal body processes are disrupted when a person fails to get enough sleep. The heart rate can vary too much, which can result in an increased risk of heart diseases, such as atherosclerosis and hypertension. The production of new red blood cells are compromised without enough sleep. The immune system doesn't function optimally. Muscle pain and muscle tremors may occur due to mineral imbalances. Metabolic disorders, which can be caused by disruption in the normal secretion of hormones, can develop in the long run.

Studies show an increased risk of type 2 diabetes, obesity and growth suppression for people who are frequently deprived of sleep.

Someone who fails to get enough sleep becomes easily irritable and stressed. An irritable and stressed person tends to eat more on immediate need, so he or she may eat too much, not enough, or irregularly. These poor eating habits can make the hormones insulin and glucagon levels fluctuate as a result. In particular, altered insulin sensitivity develops with poor eating habits.

Biologically, the hormone ghrelin, which stimulates appetite, increases for a person who is deprived of sleep. The hormone leptin, which signals the brain to induce a feeling of satiety, decreases. This causes a person to eat more than what he or she actually needs. Since the leptin levels are down, cravings for high sugar or high fat foods increase, while the feeling of satiety is not easily achieved. This contributes to unhealthy eating patterns and imbalances in nutrition which can later escalate into diabetes, obesity, or other health problems.

When the body perceives stress levels rising, it responds by storing fat, resulting in a higher fat build up and ultimately higher body mass overall. Storing fat is the body's response, instead of burning these stores; for cellular repair and recovery, a process which is optimized during sleep.

Caffeine and other stimulants can help with the immediate effects of sleep deprivation, like the lack of concentration and daytime sleepiness, but only temporarily. Unfortunately, they do not work to prevent long term consequences, and dependence on them during the day can further disrupt good sleep at night.

Eventually, we need to give up the coffee buzz and catch up on our beauty rest instead.

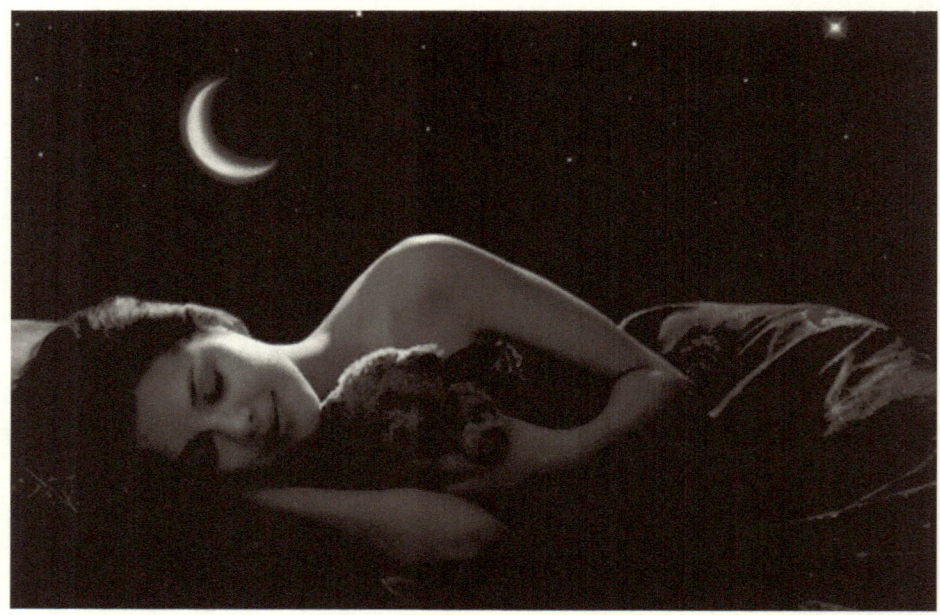

The Science of Sleep

"There is a time for many words, and there is also a time for sleep." -Homer, *The Odyssey*

Sleep is more than just a needed habit. It is more than just a hunger of the body for energy. It is more than an unexplained ritual that leads to the realm of dreams. Although sleep still remains mysterious in a sense, breakthroughs are progressively being achieved in our methodical attempts to discover more about it, thanks to the study of the wonders of sleep.

Think about these questions: How does sleep arrive? How does it take over the human senses? How does the brain descend into sub-consciousness, only to be roused later at a certain time? What do we actually know about sleep?

To gain a deeper understanding of the mechanisms involved during sleep, we will be talking about the occurrence, stages, and duration of sleep. We will be delving into the details: the science of sleep.

Occurrence of Sleep

How does sleep happen? How do we actually "go to sleep"? Sleep occurs and is controlled by three factors: the circadian clock, the sleep-wake homeostasis, and willed behavior.

The circadian clock is a built-in and self-sustained body clock, that governs our biological functions in a 24 hour cycle. It is located in the hypothalamus, as a distinct group of cells called the suprachiasmatic nuclei (SCN). The suprachiasmatic nuclei create a person's sleep-wake schedule. These cells work by receiving information about the amount of surrounding light coming through the eyes. The retina of the eyes typically contain photoreceptors, which are the rods and cones for vision, and ganglion cells that are light sensitive. In particular, these ganglion cells project directly to the suprachiasmatic nuclei, which take in the amount of light that is in the environment, then use it to interpret the length of "day time" and "night time".

The presence of sunlight and artificial light are important in establishing the sleep-wake rhythm in this process. Studies have shown that the presence of artificial light, such as fluorescent lamps and light from electronic devices delay the onset of sleep. Time zones also play a part in maintaining this rhythm, as seen among frequent travelers like pilots, flight stewards and stewardesses. Since they change time zones frequently, their concept of day and night becomes disrupted, so they can get fatigued more easily than those who remain in a single time zone.

After the suprachiasmatic nuclei interpret the length of day and night, they transmit this information to the pineal gland. The pineal gland secretes the hormone melatonin, which is one of the circadian markers that help establish the sleep-wake rhythm in the circadian clock. During the day, this hormone is present in nearly undetectable levels in our bodies. At night around 9pm it increases, especially in the absence of light.

Another crucial factor in establishing our sleep-wake cycle is core body temperature, which is also considered a circadian marker. The circadian clock can cause the core body temperature to lower, especially when it is time to sleep. Our core body temperature is typically at its lowest point at around 5AM, which is 2 hours before the commonly established wake-up time when the sun rises.

The circadian clock is also known to work with other enzymes and hormones like adenosine, which promotes the feeling of sleepiness. It is also responsible for determining the time when the body wakes up.

The sleep-wake homeostasis works in balance with the circadian clock, by communicating to the body that it needs sleep. This switch is dependent on the need of the body to rest. This is directly related to the overall condition of the body. If a person is slightly sleep deprived, he or she will generally wake up at a certain hour, and not be able to sleep again because of the circadian rhythm.

Willed behavior is one aspect that is exclusive to humans, as they have higher brain function and decision making ability. It profoundly affects a person's sleeping habits. For example, a night worker can habitually choose to wake up at 10PM, work his eight hour shift, head home just as the sun is rising, and sleep at 8AM. The body will need to adjust to these demands, and with that the circadian clock and the sleep-wake homeostasis follow through as needed. From here we can see that work schedules and activities of daily life are major factors that can affect sleeping patterns.

Stages of Sleep

The stages of sleep were first studied and hypothesized by Alfred Lee Loomis and his colleagues in 1939. It was typically assessed using polysomnography in a sleep laboratory. EEG of brain waves, EOG of eye movements, and EMG of skeletal muscle activity were recorded as part of the assessment.

Sleep is divided into two types: REM and non-REM. REM means rapid eye movement. It is the stage when the brain is more active and dreams occur. Non-REM, which is also called delta sleep or slow wave sleep, is divided into three stages: N1, N2, and N3. Non-REM sleep is referred to as the deep restorative sleep phase. Commonly, one sleep cycle starts with N1, followed by N2, then N3, and ends with the REM stage. This cycle lasts for approximately 90 minutes and repeats itself about four to six times a night. The amount of time a person spends in each sleep stage varies throughout the night. Most deep sleep takes place early in the first half of the night. Later, after the fourth sleep cycle, the REM stage becomes longer and alternates with the N2 phase.

N1 is the stage between sleep and wakefulness; the transition into sleep. This lasts about five minutes. The muscles are still active and the eyes roll slowly with moderate opening and closing. Wakefulness is still easily achieved with slight external stimuli.

N2 is the stage where the person sleeping is eventually difficult to rouse by external stimuli; the light sleep phase. This lasts for about ten to twenty-five minutes. Physical movement stops. The heart rate, breathing rate, and pulse rate all slow down. The core body temperature also decreases.

N3 is the stage when the person cannot easily be stimulated to wakefulness; the deep sleep phase. This is the deepest phase of sleep, and if a person is awakened at this point, he or she will be disoriented and groggy for a few minutes. Blood flow is directed away from the brain and to the muscles for restoration and repair.

REM stage was discovered by Eugene Aserinsky using the EEG around 1950. It is the stage when the sleeping person's voluntary muscles (for example, your arm and leg muscles) are paralyzed. This stage of sleep, is reached after about 70 to 90 minutes after initially falling asleep, is activated by acetylcholine and inhibited by serotonin. Rapid eye movement stage is also called paradoxical sleep, because this is the stage where the person is the most difficult to rouse, but the EEG waves exhibit brain activity that is similar to wakefulness. Oxygen consumption by the brain is significantly higher at this stage. REM sleep is also known as the dream sleep phase because this is the stage when dreams may occur.

A normal adult spends about 50% of sleeping time in N2 stage, 20% in REM, and 30% in the other stages of sleep. Quality does count when it comes to sleep. The two most important stages of sleep are the N3 (or the deep sleep phase) and the REM stage.

N3 phase is the time when the body is renewed. Notably, the damaging effects of sleep deprivation are from the lack of deep sleep (N3 phase). Why is this so? Most of the growth, development, and repair processes of the body happen in this stage. Getting deep sleep at night allows us to wake up feeling refreshed and energized. It enables us to move productively throughout the day.

REM phase is when the mind is renewed. In REM sleep, the brain replenishes its stock of neurotransmitters like serotonin and dopamine which contributes to having a good mood during the day. In this stage, everything a person encounters in the day, is processed to form connections that enhance memory and learning.

Human growth hormone (or HGH) is also produced during sleep as well as during exercise. It is produced by the pituitary gland and aids in increasing glucose uptake in muscle cells, helping synthesis in the liver and muscles and is responsible for breaking down fat.

Because of these functions, HGH increases fat burning and diminishes fat storage leading to an overall leaner body.

HGH is produced more in the earlier hours of the night than the later hours. For this reason, it's better to sleep from 10PM - 7AM, rather than midnight to 8AM. This makes a strong case for an earlier bedtime.

Another reason to opt for an earlier bedtime is to avoid a second wind of energy that can hit somewhere between 10 - 11PM for many people. When this 'second wind' comes, it can make getting to sleep difficult as well. The best strategy to cope with that is to get to sleep before it hits, and get the benefits of maximum HGH production.

Duration of Sleep

So how much sleep is required to be healthy? According to the National Institute of Health, adults (18 years old and up) need about 7.5 to 9 hours of sleep a night, and teenagers (12 to 18 years old) need 8.5 to 10 hours of sleep.

School age children (5 to 12 years old) need 10 to 11 hours of sleep, preschoolers (3 to 5 years old) need 11 to 13 hours of sleep, and toddlers (1 to 3 years old) need 12 to 14 hours of sleep. Infants (3 months to 1 year old) need 14-15 hours of sleep.

Although people try to adapt to getting less sleep than they need, they do not truly succeed because sleep is a universal necessity that is vital for human survival. The duration of sleep also increases for a person who is sick or who has been deprived of sleep. Among the elderly, studies have shown that the depth of sleep is less, and the length of sleep is shorter. This explains why the elderly tend to get up at earlier hours in the morning, and are more easily awakened with external stimuli.

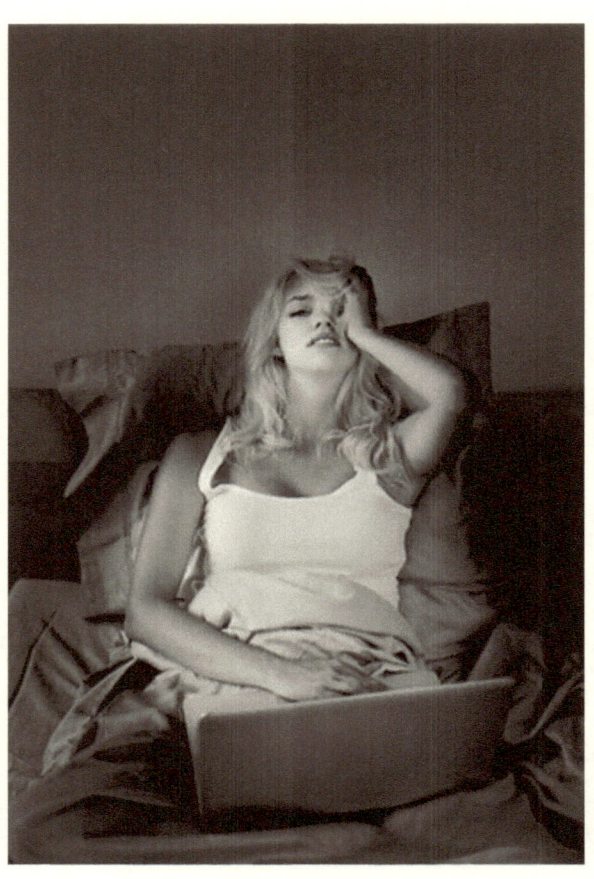

The Dilemma with Insomnia

Sleep deprivation is defined as the lack of sleep due to the lack of opportunity or time to sleep because of voluntary choices. It is not being able to sleep because of personally choosing not to sleep in order to make way for other activities or existing priorities. As discussed in the introduction, it is a widespread problem nowadays and is considered a public health and safety hazard. Left unaddressed, it can lead to sleep disorders.

One of the most common sleep disorder plaguing the current population is insomnia. We hear about it a lot. There's even an upbeat dance record of that title from Craig David, and it kind of makes insomnia sound fun. But for those who have experienced tossing and turning at night in bed, while the rest of the neighborhood is pleasantly dreaming away, not being able to fall asleep is far from being a fun experience.

So medically speaking, what is insomnia?

Insomnia is defined as a sleep disorder which is characterized by persistent difficulty in falling, or staying asleep as the body needs. It is also characterized by failing to get enough "quality" sleep, which means "deep, undisturbed" sleep. It is perceived as a medical sign or symptom that may be accompanied by other health issues such as psychological problems, perhaps a physical condition, or sometimes even another sleep disorder. Insomnia is commonly followed by functional impairment, as often manifested by excessive drowsiness, difficulty making decisions, inability to concentrate on daytime tasks, irritability, and delayed reaction time to stimuli. It can occur at any age, but it is particularly common among the elderly.

Now ask yourself: Do you experience difficulty in falling asleep? Do you have difficulty staying asleep? If you answered yes to both of these questions, then you are probably suffering from insomnia.

Differentiation

Sleep deprivation is not the same as insomnia. Sleep deprivation happens as an effect of voluntarily deciding to sacrifice some sleeping hours to do other things. An example would be a college student who habitually plays a game on his tablet from 11pm to 1am before finally sleeping at around 1:30am. He wakes up at 7:30am in order to make it to school for his class at 8am. That leaves about 6 hours of sleep for him to recharge.

Our personal priorities play a big role in promoting sleep deprivation. Losing even 1-2 hours of sleep at night can accumulate and greatly impact our productivity and overall health.

Insomnia, unlike sleep deprivation, is different in the sense that it is not voluntary. The time and opportunity to sleep are available for the person, but the person has difficulty doing so. Insomnia can come as a result of habitual sleep deprivation.

Symptoms

Sufferers of insomnia may be diagnosed with the following symptoms:

First, the obvious: difficulty falling asleep, which includes difficulty finding a comfortable sleeping position. The onset of sleep should be naturally achieved by the body in an average of at least 10-30 minutes, but some people experience difficulty to get into that.

Second is waking up frequently in the middle of the night and having trouble going back to sleep. This is especially true if waking up occurs in less than 6.5 hours of sleep and the person finds it hard to go back to sleep.

Third is feeling tired upon getting up in the morning, not feeling refreshed.

Irritability, general fatigue, daytime sleepiness, unexplained anxiety and problems concentrating and remembering things are also symptoms to check.

There are two kinds of insomnia according to cause: primary and secondary. Primary insomnia is not connected to any medical or psychiatric conditions. It can be caused by non-biological factors like a poor sleep schedule, a lot of noise, or too much lighting. Secondary insomnia is caused by health conditions or substance abuse, which tend to deprive the person of sleep.

There are 3 different types of insomnia according to duration: chronic, transient, and acute. The transient form lasts less than 7 days. It can be caused by a minor health problem like stress, a bout of flu, or changes to normal sleeping habits. Acute types can last for 1-3 weeks. This kind has significant impact to a person's daytime functioning ability. The chronic form of insomnia endures longer than 3 weeks, and can cause serious physiological problems such as depression, frequent mental blanks, or the development of heart disease.

Cycle of Insomnia

Insomnia has many different causes, but for the majority of the sufferers it starts with sleep deprivation.

Habitual lack of sleep encourages the brain to delay the onset of sleep and the feeling of sleepiness, which later leads to insomnia, or the difficulty of sleeping. Insomnia then results in poor sleep quality, or inadequate hours of sleep. This in turn leads to an accumulation of stress, anxiety, worry, and physical tension. These distractions decrease productivity and increase daytime sleepiness. Daytime sleepiness in particular, can promote unhealthy napping habits, which all the more contribute to insomnia.

Coping mechanisms develop as well, in attempt to manage the problem. For example, an insomniac might resort to drinking more coffee and eating more to temporarily stay awake and stay productive. To get more sleep in the evening, he or she might drink alcohol or take over-the-counter sleep medications, which might worsen the situation. The insomniac loses more sleep as the sleep rhythm is disrupted further.

Causes

Insomnia may be caused by a variety of factors. Behavioral, psychological, and medical problems are possible causes. It is important to remember that insomnia is not commonly seen as an isolated diagnosis. Usually it is perceived as a sign or symptom of an underlying health problem. In this case, it is important to get help to treat the underlying condition first, in order to treat the insomnia as well.

Behavioral and psychological problems

Psychological stress can cause insomnia. Fear, anxiety, and stress due to life experiences can possibly cause insomnia.

Major depression can be a cause of insomnia because it can result in the excessive release of the hormone called cortisol, by the hypothalamic-pituitary-adrenal axis. Excess cortisol, the stress hormone that causes wakefulness, can lead to poor sleep quality. In particular, the sufferer fails to reach N3 levels of sleep, or the realm of deep sleep, when the body is being repaired and renewed.

Among athletes, exercise induced insomnia is common. This happens when a person exercises too much. This results in a delay in the onset of sleep.

For those with night jobs and careers that require frequent travel, insomnia can also occur. Jet lag, and change in work shifts can disrupt the regular sleep pattern.

Medical problems

Physical pain due to an injury or a chronic condition like rheumatoid arthritis, can cause insomnia as well. Heartburn, digestive problems such as excessive gas or constipation, nocturnal polyuria, or excessive urination at night, can also disturb sleep.

Hormonal imbalances caused by menstruation, pregnancy, or menopause can cause insomnia.

Mental disorders such as bipolar disorder, post-traumatic stress disorder, schizophrenia, obsessive-compulsive disorder, or dementia can cause disruption in regular sleep patterns.

Substance issues

Use of stimulants in the form of herbal tea or supplements, caffeinated drinks, and cigarettes can easily rob you of well deserved sleep, especially if taken excessively.

Substance abuse in the form of alcohol, amphetamines, cocaine, methylphenidate, aripiprazole, modafinil, and even some over the counter drugs can hinder sleep. Even though alcohol is a depressant, meaning it can dull the senses and make you feel sleepy, it is a poor habit that allows you to temporarily feel sleepy, but can awaken you in the middle of the night and prevent deep sleep (N3).

Antidepressant prescription drugs and opioid pain relievers can also disrupt sleep.

What your health care provider can do

Your health care provider will ask about your sleep history and give you to a physical exam. For serious cases, you might be referred to a sleep clinic to undergo testing.

Treatment

If you are suffering from acute to chronic insomnia, it is important that you see a doctor as soon as possible in order to find the cause, especially if the underlying condition is a medical problem that needs treatment. Prevention is better than a cure, and early treatment is better than later treatment.

Mild primary insomnia can be treated in many different ways. You may simply need to modify some sleeping habits, manage your bedtime more efficiently, or check and adjust food intake as needed. Some sufferers of insomnia resort to medication immediately without consulting a physician, or without even trying non-medical solutions, which might be of more help for them by establishing good habits in the long run. Taking over the counter medications is a poor way of managing the condition because the cause of primary insomnia is usually behavioral or environmental, and if it is biological, it usually has something to do with food intake.

Medication is not mandatory. Therapy may be recommended for some, but why not try some simple methods first? You may be surprised at how easy, yet effective these tips are.

Sleep Tips

Sleep is sometimes considered a luxury, especially in current times. Frequently, it is not given the priority in our lives it deserves. Sometimes there are negative associations attached to someone who does get enough sleep and is well rested. Being deprived of it is both irritating and exhausting, and nothing takes the good out of morning faster than sleep deprivation. But there are solutions available to try at home, on your own. You might be familiar with some of them, but read on as you might find new tips as well.

Below are simple, serious solutions for those who are bent on improving their sleep and eventually, their lives. These can benefit insomniacs and non-insomniacs alike.

For the sake of better understanding, this section is divided into three main headings: Sleeping habits, bedroom management, and diet management. Since our lives make up our whole being, then from a holistic point, these tips are noticeably intertwined.

Sleeping habits

It might not seem like much at first glance, but a person's sleeping habits affect their sleeping patterns more than other factors. As mentioned earlier, one of the ways that the circadian rhythm is set, is through the person's behavioral activities throughout the day.

Here is how it works: A person who enjoys the night life tends to have sleep onset times in the wee hours of the morning, not at night. This is because his or her habit of staying up all night has already caused the brain to learn and adapt to his or her usual pattern, that of being active at a time when most people are supposed to be enjoying some well deserved sleep. Studies suggest that this disrupts the normal circadian rhythm and may cause health problems in the long run.

With that being stated, the first tip to take seriously is managing your sleep habits. How do you improve those sleep habits? Here are some tips:

1. Get an extra 30 minutes to 1 hour of sleep before you get up in the morning, for many people, this will mean going to bed a bit earlier. Since the REM stage is longer towards the end of your sleeping time, snagging an extra 30 minutes to one hour of sleep, allows you to wake up feeling more refreshed and energized. Memory and learning is enhanced in the REM stage, so you get to be

more productive throughout the day when you have enough of it. Do not oversleep, or else you might end up feeling tired.

2. Nap wisely. If done well, naps can help you recharge in the middle of the day. Such nap sessions are popularly known these days as power naps, short naps that recharge people in the daytime. But these naps may also do you harm. If overdone, naps may prevent the onset of sleep at night by disrupting your sleeping pattern.

So how do you schedule your naps properly? Take note of the sleep cycle. Have you ever experienced napping for a while, only to wake up tired later? This is because the deepest sleep occurs about 90 minutes after the onset of sleep. This is the rapid eye movement phase of sleep, and as discussed earlier, this is the time when your body consolidates memories to improve your brain's learning ability. The appropriate duration of napping should be restricted to 15 to 30 minutes only. If you sleep beyond 30 minutes, you might be awakened in the middle of the REM phase, which will cause irritation and restlessness throughout the day and sometimes even until bedtime.

3. Settle taxing activities like house chores, work related calls & tasks, eating, socializing, and other things that are stressful, about two to three hours before bed time. Your mind needs time to relax about an hour before bedtime. The night is the time to rest (unless of course you have unusual shift work). Use it well.

4. Keep a very strict sleep-wake schedule, even on weekends. This is especially helpful for insomniacs. As

the body learns its sleep-wake rhythm from habits, this is very crucial. Do not take chances on the weekend and disrupt your cycle.

5. Avoid night shifts if possible. Remember that light disrupts sleep. For insomniacs, try to get a regular work schedule to improve your performance and catch up on your sleep. If you really cannot avoid the night shift, make sure you sleep in a dark room, because it helps your brain switch to sleep mode.

6. Make sure you eat full meals at least three hours before bedtime. This will allow your body to digest properly. If you eat a heavy meal just before lying down, chances are you would feel uncomfortable, because you may feel bloated and heavy. You might find it hard to get sleep in that case.

7. Do self care rituals on time. Do not go to sleep without eating, and make sure you finish your tasks before bedtime. Are you the type who enjoys exercising or taking a bath, in order to get a good night of rest? Do them all on time, so that when it is time to sleep, you can feel relaxed and assured that you can peacefully go to sleep.

8. Schedule a bed time ritual and stick with it. If you listen to music before sleeping, go for it. If you enjoy reading, do it. If a warm bubble bath works for you, do it. It might take a few days to get used to it, but try to see what personal bedtime routine works for you. What may work for one person may not necessarily work for you.

Some experts recommend the use of two cups of Epsom salts in your bath water, and soaking in it for 20 minutes before going to bed. Studies support the use of bedtime routines as a means of allowing the body to "know" that it is almost time to go to bed. Manage your sleeping habits successfully, and you will not need to count sheep until the sun comes up.

9. Do not force yourself to sleep. Stressing yourself about sleep is not going to help. The best thing to do when you do not feel sleepy yet is to get up, sit up and walk around for about ten minutes, eat a small snack or drink milk (sleep-inducing food), then go back to bed and lie down. You can also read a book or listen to relaxing music, whatever works for you. While you are not yet sleepy, it is better to engage in relaxing activities and not to "overthink" how to get some sleep.

10. People who exercise in the morning generally sleep better than those who exercise at other times of the day or evening. This will improve blood circulation and breathing. It will also induce the feeling of tiredness later on, and help promote the onset of sleep at night.

Bedroom management

The condition of your bedroom speaks much about your personality. Is it cluttered with paperwork, gadgets, books, dirty laundry or dirty plates? Is it dim or bright? Does it contain a lot of electronics like the television, or computer? It is important to look into the element of your physical bedroom surroundings, if you are serious about improving your sleep quality. The bedroom is the sleeper's haven, and it can impact greatly the depth and quality of your sleep.

According to the National Sleep Foundation, the ideal room for sleeping in, is a room that is cool, dark, and quiet. With that knowledge, here are some tips:

1. Make sure that you turn off the room lights because the dark activates the production of melatonin and it tells your brain that it is time to go to sleep. If you are not used to it, then maybe this is the time to change that.

2. Even a little light can delay the onset of sleep, so it would be good for you to switch off your night lights, and put away your electronic gadgets. Yes, you can live without your mobile phones and tablets for a few hours of well deserved sleep. Studies have suggested that gadgets pose a threat to your sleep and health, though there are no conclusive findings yet. Have you ever experienced sleeping with your cell phone beside you in

bed? There may be a tendency to feel very tired after that. We do not know exactly why, according to research at this point, but it might have something to do with the radiation emitted by various electronic equipment.

It is safe to say that the light emitted by the screens can delay the feeling of sleepiness, so if you can put it out of your sight, then that would be helpful for you.

3. Remember that the body's core temperature tends to decrease during sleep, so it will be helpful to adjust room temps and bedding to account for that.

4. Activities like eating food, chatting with friends, and working, should be restricted as much as possible, to the

living room and other parts of the house. This will help you get used to the bedroom as being the right environment that is conducive for your rest.

5. Make sure that you are using the right kind of mattress, pillow, and blanket. This depends on your preferences, so try to find what works best for you. Do you like fluffy pillows more than flat ones? Do you like a hard mattress or a bouncy bed? Do you like fleece or cotton blankets? Discover, adjust, and test it out. If you have the budget then you should go ahead and buy replacements as needed.

A good night's sleep is priceless, because your life depends on it. Think of it this way: if you sleep well, you will be more productive. If you become more productive, you get more tasks done. If you get more tasks done, you can have that edge in your career and have a greater opportunity to earn more.

6. Change your linens frequently. Fresh linens are comforting after a long hard day. As well as the linens, you should make sure the room is clean and uncluttered, so that it will be pleasant and tranquil to be in your room.

7. If you need extra pillows or an ergonomic mattress, do that so you can get a good night's rest. Your health and productivity will tell you, that these things can really pay off in the long run.

8. Some people sleep well with music or some type of white noise. Others don't. Choose whatever works for

you, but sometimes silence can be the best way to invite sleep.

9. Your sleepwear (or not), is important. Make sure it helps keep you the right temperature while sleeping, and that it is comfortable for you.

10. Keep pets off the bed. This is especially needed if you are awakened by its movement or noises. The bedroom is yours for recharging, and you have to put a priority on your sleep. You can make your pet its own special and cozy sleeping place.

11. Use extra accessories as necessary. If you have a noisy neighborhood, use earplugs. If you have extra light coming from the outside, use an eye mask. If you need a

huggable pillow or stuffed toy to sleep, go ahead. The bedroom is your own haven, make it yours!

12. Make your bedroom a place you love to be in. Some studies suggest that the color blue is the most conducive for sleep. Have some live indoor plants in your room. The oxygen they produce is helpful, they are beautiful and give a fresh scent to the room. As often as possible, allow fresh air into your bedroom.

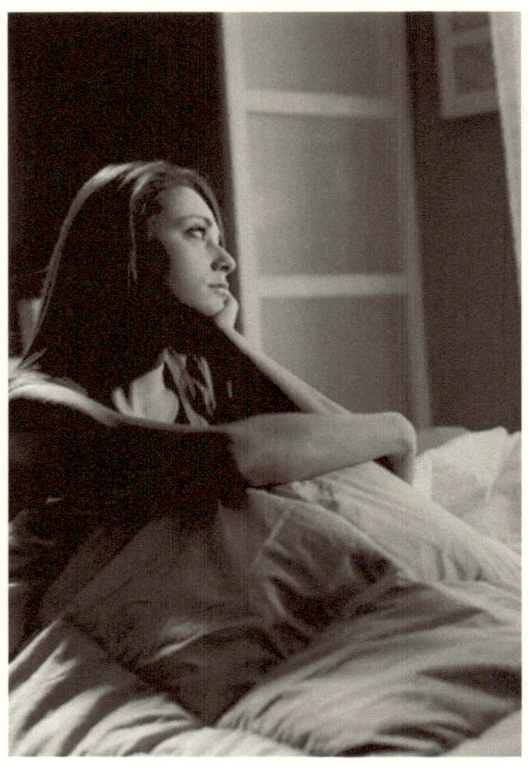

Diet management

Theories have long abounded that our food intake is one of the factors that either enable sleep, or cause it to escape from us. It is important that we delve further into this topic, and modify our diets as needed. Here are some useful tips:

Stop Losing Sleep

1. Avoid smoking and drinking in the evening. Alcoholic drinks, being a depressant, allow for light sleep, but not deep sleep. It has a 'rebound' effect of preventing sleep later in the night. It also may cause you get up at night due to a full bladder, headache, or stomach ache.

2. Avoid smoking two to three hours before bedtime. Cigarettes are stimulants which cause your brain to be alert, so it delays the onset of sleep.

3.   Limit your consumption of coffee and other caffeinated drinks. Caffeine is a stimulant which alerts your brain, thereby preventing the onset of sleep. It is wise to limit your intake to one cup of coffee a day, and that being in the morning hours. If it still keeps you awake at night, it is better to quit altogether, or switch to decaf.   According to experts, if you are a coffee

drinker, you should have your last serving of coffee just before noon. Ideally you should have a maximum of two cups of coffee per day, if you can manage it.

4. Avoid drinking too much liquid a couple hours before bedtime, especially if you are the type who frequently feels the need to urinate.

5. Eat tryptophan rich food items in the early evening. Milk is the all-time classic example of this, and it has been on top of the list of the popular remedies, for those who find it hard to get to sleep. Multiple studies and research have proven that a glass of milk before bedtime helps the body get into the sleep zone. Other examples of tryptophan rich foods are cottage cheese, cashew nuts, chicken, turkey, soybeans, and tuna.

Exploring Sleep Cures

"The main facts in human life are five: birth, food, sleep, love, and death." -E.M. Forster

This chapter about sleep cures has been intentionally written separately from the diet management and sleeping habits sections, so that you can explore the suggestions and choose easily for yourself those that suit you. Some of these are classic home remedies that have been around for a long time. Others are newer natural alternative treatments to try.

There are synthetic treatments that can be purchased without a prescription. It is advisable to consult a physician to get professional advice, before testing them on your own. To find out more about the popular sleep treatments available today, read on:

Melatonin

Melatonin is a naturally occurring hormone in the body that is produced by the pineal gland in the brain. It induces sleep by causing drowsiness and lowering the central body temperature. Normally, the level of melatonin rises from mid to late evening, and it drops in the early hours of the morning. The production of melatonin decreases as people age. Because it is a hormone, it might not be for everyone however.

Melatonin supplements are taken by mouth in the form of capsules, tablets, or liquid suspensions. They are also available in sublingual tablets and transdermal patches. It is used to treat many medical conditions. A common use is when it's used to treat insomnia by prolonging sleep. According to studies, it is safe to take in low doses for short term use of up to 3 months. But no research for long term use has provided evidence that it is safe to use beyond 3 months. Research has yet to support its use for other sleep disorders, so it should not be treated as a one pill wonder.

Side effects and Contraindications

Melatonin supplements can cause minimal side effects if taken according to a doctor's advice. Some unwanted side effects may include nausea, irritability, a decrease in body temperature, groggy feeling in the morning, and minor changes in blood pressure. It is also not recommended for those who have heart conditions, liver problems, diabetes and autoimmune disorders. This should be taken with caution by those who regularly drive and operate heavy machinery.

Tryptophan

Tryptophan is an amino acid that promotes normal growth & development and nitrogen balance. It is derived from specific foods that contain it. It is used by the body to produce niacin (vitamin B3) and serotonin, which is a key hormone in the sleep-wake cycle. In order for tryptophan to be converted to niacin, the body needs to have enough iron, riboflavin (vitamin B2), and pyridoxine (vitamin B6).

Tryptophan is naturally available in most protein rich foods. It is found in dried dates, chocolate, red meat, bananas, oats, milk, cheese, sesame seeds, yogurt, turkey, chicken, peanuts, eggs, fish, pumpkin seeds, sunflower seeds, soy, other types of nuts and tofu.

Tryptophan supplements are taken orally and have long been known to induce sleep as evidenced by clinical research results in the late 1970s. It has been shown to be effective in improving the quality of sleep. It decreases the time needed to fall asleep and increases the total amount of sleep time. These desirable effects are best displayed among those with mild insomnia and those who had difficulty with falling asleep. However, it is not recommended for chronic insomnia.

Side effects and Contraindications

Tryptophan supplements can cause side effects like heartburn, gastric irritation, belching, nausea, diarrhea, and loss of appetite. It is also not recommended for pregnant and breastfeeding women, and people who suffer from digestive problems, liver disease, kidney disease, diabetes, and blood disorders. Caution should also be taken by users who drive or operate heavy machinery.

5-HTP

5-Hydroxytryptophan is a naturally occurring amino acid that is part of the biosynthesis of melatonin and tryptophan. It is available in capsule form and is used as a supplement to manage insomnia. It works by increasing the production of serotonin which helps re-establish healthy sleep-wake patterns for sufferers of insomnia. And because serotonin's metabolic processes lead to an increase in melatonin levels, it greatly helps insomniacs get their good nights of sleep. Some studies even suggest that it is better than tryptophan supplements in inducing sleep, because it has very minimal to no side effects. But that is also the problem with this supplement; it has been criticized for its lack of research to back up its effectiveness.

Side effects and Contraindications

The side effects to watch out for are similar to that of tryptophan supplements. Possible side effects are heartburn, gastric irritation, belching, nausea, diarrhea, and loss of appetite. Caution should also be taken by users who drive or operate heavy machinery. More research is needed to establish these findings.

Kyle Richards

Valerian Root

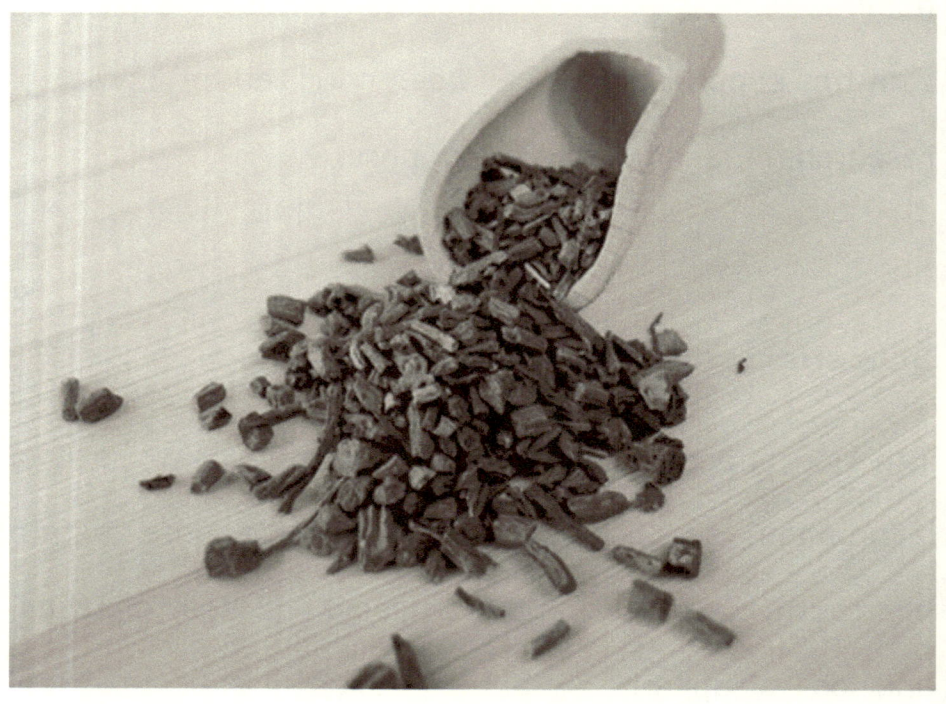

Valerian root is one of the best known natural sleep aids. The sedative root extract is available in the form of capsules, tea supplements, and even oils. It is also one of the oldest remedies around, as it has been used for its calming effects since the 1800s. According to research, it works to hasten the onset of sleep, and is supported by studies. Some experts recommend taking it with a melatonin supplement to improve its effectiveness, especially among the elderly who naturally produce less melatonin.

Side effects and Contraindications

Valerian root supplements can cause headaches, morning grogginess, excitability, and even insomnia in some people. It is also not recommended for pregnant and breastfeeding women. Caution should be taken by users who drive or operate heavy machinery. This is not recommended for people who are suffering from liver or kidney disease. This should not be taken by people who are scheduled for surgery within two weeks, because it can affect the effects of anesthesia and other medications commonly used during surgery.

Chamomile Tea

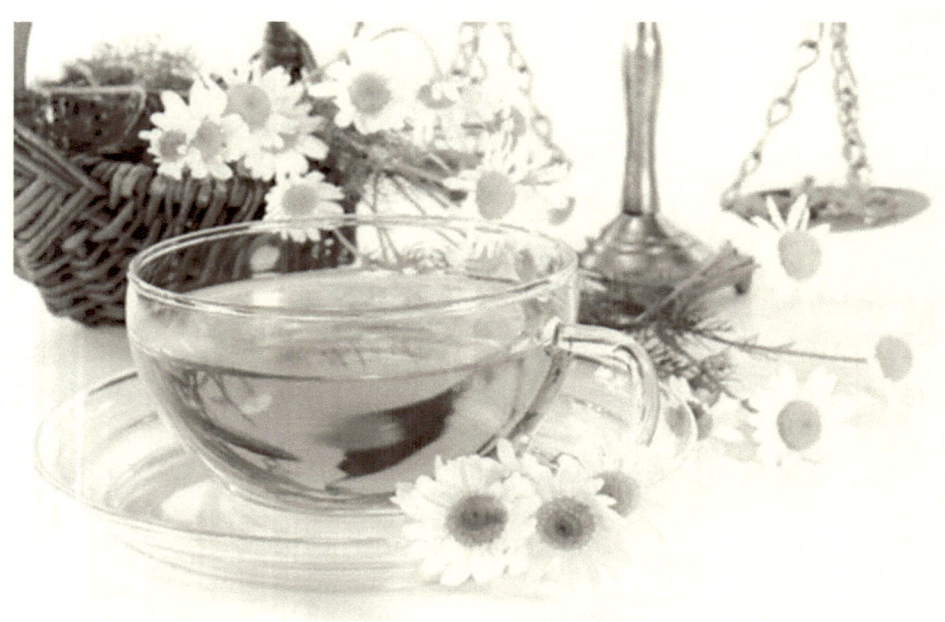

Chamomile tea is also known as the night time tea, thanks to its mild sedative effect that has been known about for centuries. Generally considered safe, this herbal tea has a reputation of promoting sleepiness, as well as easing anxiety and depression. Two specific types of chamomile are especially noted for their health benefits: German chamomile and Roman chamomile.

Although drinking chamomile tea is a popular choice for those who want to get a good night's sleep, there are only limited studies to back up its effectiveness. Still, a warm cup of tea can help you relax your senses and is soothing, right before bedtime. Be careful not to drink too much, though, or a full bladder may disturb your sleep.

Cherry Juice

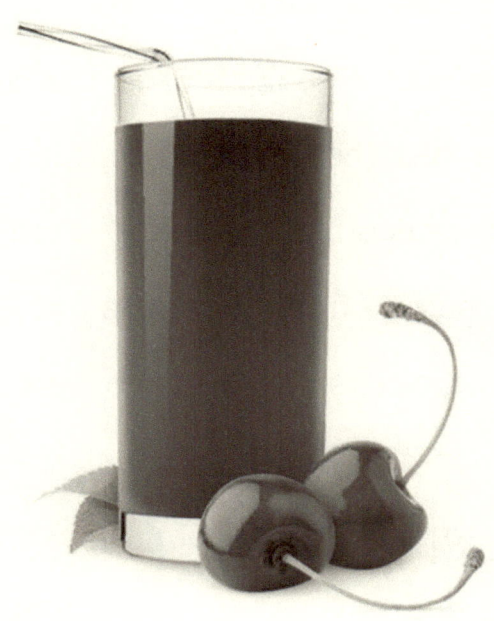

Tart cherry juice seems promising as a sleep aid. In a short term clinical study, experts concluded that drinking two one ounce servings of this juice improved the quality of sleep among the participants. They napped less and had longer sleep periods. They also had significantly increased melatonin levels. Note that melatonin helps in the regulation of the sleep-wake cycle.

Also, a recent study presented at the American Society of Nutrition's annual meeting affirms the effectiveness of tart cherry juice. They believe that it is indeed an effective and preferable treatment especially for the elderly who suffer from insomnia. It is an easily recommended choice, since tart cherry juice is safer than other sleep aids that have potential side effects. The researchers also found some compounds in tart cherries that could prevent the breakdown of tryptophan, which is a possible key to its effectiveness in promoting better quality of sleep.

Pumpkin Powder

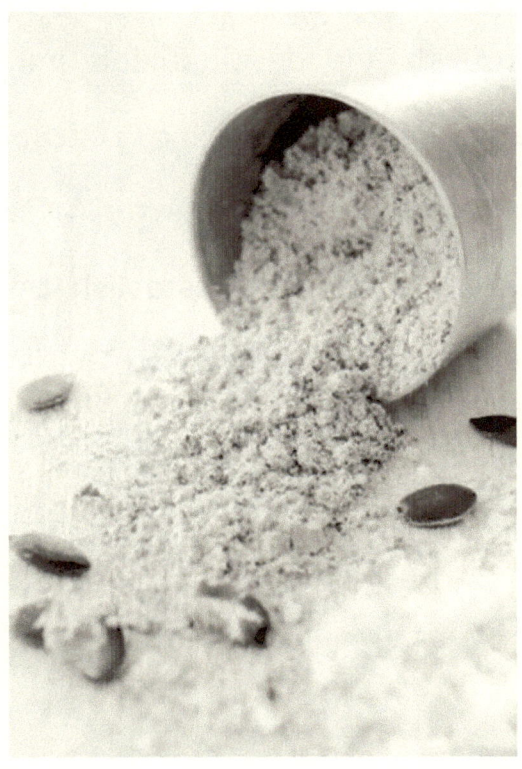

Pumpkin is known to be rich in vitamin A and B. But recently the seeds are becoming popular as a natural food supplement in order to help people sleep. Pumpkin powder is derived from ground pumpkin seeds. They are known to contain high levels of tryptophan, which improves the onset of sleep. In particular, the World

Health Organization advocates the consumption of pumpkin seeds for its high zinc content. Aside from maintaining growth and development, immune support and male sexual function, zinc contributes to the production of serotonin and melatonin, two important neurotransmitters which help establish the sleep-wake rhythm in our brains. It is also a rich source of magnesium which contributes to proper blood flow and production of energy. It contains antioxidants which promotes cell rejuvenation and recovery.

Pumpkin powder is indeed a potent ingredient with many benefits in addition to inducing relaxation and sleep. It is preferred not only as a natural cure over prescription pills for insomniacs, but also for its many other health benefits. According to some experts, pumpkin powder is best taken with carbohydrates to increase its effectiveness. The simplest way to ingest it is to mix one or two teaspoons of pumpkin powder in warm milk and drink it about an hour before bedtime.

Recently, pumpkin powder promoters are coming up with organic supplements that are available in powder and snack bar forms. Some of them have created flavored powder that can be mixed with water. These are relatively new in the market at this point, so only limited clinical testing has been done. Even so, many people are buying these products in health stores as a means to alleviate insomnia.

Supplements can be used to manage insomnia. They work differently for everyone. Again it is wise to consult your trusted medical practitioner before you decide to take any of these. Natural and safe alternatives are becoming more preferred by people for their effectiveness without the side effects.

Magnesium

Magnesium is a mineral that is powerful for helping to fight stress and anxiety. It helps relax tight muscles, calm the nervous system and reduce pain. It also helps regulate blood sugar levels and blood pressure.

It is believed that the majority of people are getting insufficient quantities of magnesium in their diets. Even a small lack of magnesium can affect sleep quality. An effective way to improve your sleep is adding magnesium rich foods into your diet. Some good ones are pumpkin seeds, wheat germ, almonds and green leafy vegetables. See medical advice however before taking the supplement form, as it may interact with medications you may currently be taking.

Conclusion

Thank you for taking the time to read this book. The goal of it was to raise awareness about the importance of sleep, the consequences of sleep deprivation, and available solutions for sufferers of sleep deprivation. Perhaps it has encouraged you to seek medical help. If you feel that this has provided information and new options for you to try, then it has accomplished its purpose.

It is our hope that you find real solutions to improve your sleep, gain more energy and have optimum health!

If you enjoyed this book or received value from it in any way, would you be kind enough to leave a review for this book on Amazon? Thank you!

www.ingramcontent.com/pod-product-compliance
Lightning Source LLC
Chambersburg PA
CBHW050419290526
45786CB00003B/1321